I0440643

Ageless Skin

New anti-aging secrets for younger, beautiful, radiant skin

by Paula Hawley
AgelessSkinSecrets.com

Introduction

Perfect skin is not a miracle, it's a process – and YOU can have the recipe!

We all want glowing, radiant skin no matter what our age, but the anti-aging and beauty business is a multi-billion dollar industry with an overwhelming sea of products. With all the skin care options on the market today, it's easy to feel overwhelmed by all the choices.

Is there a way to make wrinkles actually disappear without Botox?

Do brands endorsed by Hollywood doctors really work?

Are antioxidants the next true anti-aging breakthrough?

Which products are really worth your money and your time?

Here are a few things you'll get from this book:

- Expand your knowledge of helpful skincare products – based on science, not hype
- Understand the difference between healthy and harmful ingredients
- Find natural skincare solutions that offer real results and save you money
- Gain a basic understanding of your skin and its function
- Discover how to take better care of yourself for ageless, radiant skin

Table of Contents

Radiant Skin From The Outside In

It's true that genuine beauty radiates from the inside out. Supporting our skin from the outside helps us like what we see reflected in our mirror, giving us more confidence to allow our spirit and true beauty to really shine through.

Basic skin care

Cleansing and moisturizing are non-negotiable daily skin care rituals. Exfoliating, toning, and other treatments or special salon services are add-ons that depend on your skin type and other variables.

Here's a personal story:

When I was a teenager, my mother started harping on me to wash my face twice a day and use a moisturizer, and always in an upward motion. She told me specifically to apply moisturizer around the eye area very gently by lightly patting with the pad of the ring finger (it's the weakest finger). She said this because when she was working as a nurse, one of her patients who was 92 years old with beautiful skin had shared this as her "secret".

Since I was a fairly ugly pre-teen and still feeling the sting of many peer insults, I heeded this advice as often as possible, and have continued to this day. My younger sister, however, ignored this advice and now gets a bit irritated that most people think she is the older, rather than the younger of the two of us!

Cleansing

It's most important to wash your face every night, with warm (not hot) water, so that pores don't become clogged with make-up, dirt, environmental debris, and the daily buildup of sebum (our natural oil) that has made its way to the surface.

Water-proof makeup will need to be removed with a gentle makeup remover before cleansing your face. A cotton pad with a few drops of olive oil is inexpensive and most effective. Using a nubby washcloth or battery-operated facial cleansing brush adds a bit of the exfoliation step into your cleansing process.

Now the eternal question of cleanser vs. soap: Personally, I've always been a soap and water girl. It gets the job done, quick and easy. Over the years I've found that most bar soaps from the drug store are too harsh on facial skin. Now I look for olive oil or glycerin (glycerin is a natural humectant, meaning it attracts moisture from the air to your skin) based soaps such as Purpose Gentle Cleansing Bar with glycerin, Olivella, Kiss My Face, or something interesting from the local health food store. Definitely leave the deodorant bars for use only on the parts that need deodorizing.

The market for facial cleansers and body washes has mushroomed over recent years.
Cleansers tend to be pricier, but may be gentler on your skin due to a lower pH than bar soap. The cleansing process is brief, so whatever you choose to use won't be on your skin for long anyway. When making your choice, whether you choose bar soap, liquid soap, cleanser for your face or a body wash for the rest of you, reading labels is the best way to guide your decision-making process (see the Ingredient Watchlist below).

Here is a list of common skin irritants you should avoid in any skin care product:

- Sodium lauryl sulfate, Sodium laureth sulfate
- Parabens (Butyllparaben Propylparaben, Methylparaben, Ethylparaben)
- DEA (diethanolamine), MEA (monoethanolamine), TEA (treiethanolamine)
- Mineral oil, paraffin, propylene glycol, butylene glycol, isopropyl alcohol, petrolatum, isopropyl alcohol, SD alcohol 40, ethyl alcohol
- Fragrance (indicating an artificial fragrance rather than a natural fruit or plant extract or essential oil blend)
- Triclosan

Toning

Toning is not necessary, but is a step that's often included in skincare rituals. The purpose of a toner is to remove the last traces of makeup and daily grime and/or to act as a chemical exfoliant. Most toners on the market are primarily rubbing alcohol, which can be very drying and irritating to skin. Some contain witch hazel, a natural astringent, and salicylic acid. If your skin is extremely oily you may find that a toner helps, but you'll still need to use a light moisturizer afterward.

Exfoliation

When it comes to keeping skin fitting well and looking great, and you're already eating right, exercising and hydrating, regular exfoliation ramps up your results naturally. Since the outer layer of our skin is made up of flattened, dead skin cells, we can help bring a fresher look and smoother feel to our skin by intentionally exfoliating in order to speeding up the natural shedding process. Be gentle with this, though, because heavy-handed exfoliation can cause skin irritation or damage.

Daily washing with a clean washcloth and the soap or cleanser of your choice is the simplest way to exfoliate your face and your body. However, it may be too rough for sensitive skin and incomplete for promoting a smoother skin texture. I'm still waiting for Santa Claus to bring me something fancier than a washcloth. Many of my friends though, swear by their battery powered brush devices, like Clarisonic, for deep cleansing and exfoliating.

Exfoliating gloves are the latest trendy item in the beauty isle, and they sure make it easy to scrub-a-dub-dub. Best results come with a gentle pressure and circular motion when you're scrubbing with these.

It is wise to steer clear of loofahs because they tend to harbor bacteria. And even if you have an antimicrobial net buff puff you should consider regular replacement (much like you would a toothbrush).

Dry brushing your extremities and trunk just prior to a shower is extremely helpful for managing dry, flaky skin. It also helps increase circulation. Look for a body brush with natural bristles on a wooden handle (I found mine at Bed, Bath & Beyond). Start at your feet and work up your legs (toward your heart) and torso with gentle, short, brisk strokes. Then start at the back of your hands working up your arms. I like to do this standing in the dry tub or shower so that the dead skin can be easily rinsed down the drain.

Scrubs are great to use weekly (less often if your skin is super sensitive). There are oodles of body scrubs on the market in every price range you care to explore. Recent articles in several beauty-focused magazines recommend avoiding scrubs that contain granules from nuts or plastic beads because these have the potential to tear or abrade your skin.

For scrubs, the best choices are based around salt or sugar. Sugar is slightly less abrasive than salt, so keep that in mind if your skin tends to be sensitive. These types of scrubs are easy to find in any store that carries healthy and beauty items. Even better, it is super easy to make your own.

Here is a simple recipe guide:

Get a wide-mouth container with a lid so you can make enough to store for a few uses. Mix together 1 cup of salt or sugar (the basic table size granules of either) and 1/2 cup of oil. They will not likely to stay mixed so stir it up often.

I recommend using either olive oil or extra virgin coconut oil. Coconut oil will be easier to mix up during the summer months than in the winter because it's liquid above about 75 degrees and solid below 75 degrees. Even if you mix it up in the summer and want to use it when it's solidified in the winter months, it'll soften as soon as it hits your skin.

Other popular oils to use include sweet almond oil (a massage industry favorite due to its viscosity), safflower oil, or other vegetable oil. These tend to turn rancid fairly quickly, so make small batches if you use these oils. Definitely avoid using mineral oil (this includes baby oil) because of its petroleum basis.

Skin really LOVES olive oil, so that's my choice. But I don't like smelling like an olive so I like to add 2 to 5 drops of essential oil to my mix. Not all essential oils smell great with olive oil, but lavender, mint, or rosemary are good choices. Rose essential oil has a long history in skin care due to its moisturizing, antiseptic, and anti-inflammatory properties as well as its ability to refine skin texture and help heal wounds.

For more advanced exfoliation methods you would need to schedule with a clinical aesthetician through a med-spa or dermatologist center to receive treatments like glycolic or alphahydroxy peels, microdermabrasion and other medical-grade services.

Smoothing Rough Areas

Feet often need extra attention. Callouses and corns are a build-up of skin as a response to pressure or friction that can end up creating pain and even disrupt your ability to walk comfortably. Corns are thickened areas that occur between the toes or on a joint. Callouses tend to form most often in the heel area or ball of the foot as a response to extra pressure from long periods of standing, poorly fitted shoes, dry skin, or walking barefooted.

Hands may also develop callouses with repeated handling of objects that create pressure in specific areas (like gardening tools or sports and fitness equipment). Wearing gloves when gardening or lifting weights and wearing properly fitted shoes with a wide toe box can help avoid the formation of callouses or corns.

If you're experiencing pain or bleeding as a result of severe callousing, you should consult with your doctor for treatment and to be sure there's not an underlying cause. For home treatment of minor callouses and corns, a pumice stone is the old fashioned standard tool for removing the rough build-up. The pumice should be used on pre-soaked, still damp skin to gently rub away the thick, rough skin.

Some people try using a "cheese grater" device, but that is a good way to injure the fresh, healthy skin underneath the callous. For very thick callouses, dermatologists and salon pedicure services may offer a razoring technique to remove heavy callouses. Never try to cut or razor a callous or corn yourself!

My personal preference for callous abatement is a kinder and gentler sandpaper foot file with a medium grit on one side and a fine grit on the other. With gentle pressure on dry feet, you can buff away the roughness before showering.

Moisturizing feet is best done at night, just before tucking them under the covers. That way the moisturizer has all night to absorb and you won't be struggling to keep from sliding out of your shoes all day. Be sure to clean your feet before applying moisturizer, and if you're prone to getting up in the night you will want to put on a pair of cotton socks to avoid slipping on your way to the potty.

Moisturizing

All cleansing products, whether you choose soap or liquid cleanser, strip oils from your skin's surface in the process of cleansing. If they didn't, they wouldn't get your face clean. So, once your face has been relieved of its daily accumulation of grime, applying a light moisturizer helps to sort of reassure your skin that all is well and it does not need to ramp up the production of natural oils to make up for what has just been removed.

Often, when oily skin is routinely cleansed and lightly moisturized it becomes more balanced and less prone to breakouts. Naturally dry skin may benefit from a heavier moisturizer, or even a small amount of extra virgin coconut oil or extra virgin olive oil.

Anti-Aging Night Treatment

Some products contain ingredients that are best used at night, because some of the best anti-aging ingredients break down quickly in sunlight. Plus, your body is in a naturally healing state during sleep. So using a rejuvenating or anti-aging treatment at night enhances that restorative and regenerative cycle.

How to Tighten Skin Naturally

Getting Fit

We all know (and hear often) about the importance of exercise for maintaining optimum health. It makes sense that getting in gear can also benefit your skin. Building muscle to replace fat will give the appearance of tighter skin due to the greater firmness of muscle tissue versus the flabby softness of fat.

A brisk walk or a jog can bring an instant glow to your skin. Exercise is one of the best ways to nourish your skin cells, and sweating cleans out your pores. Getting your heart pumping increases circulation, which sends more oxygen to the skin. This encourages cell renewal and helps to detoxify your entire system, effectively cleansing your skin from the inside.

Battling Cellulite: Firming and Contouring

If you still find yourself with dimply, saggy or baggy skin and don't want to resort to invasions of scalpels, suction wands or other scary gadgets, there are now some effective alternatives.
Some spas offer expensive options like "Fat Freezing" and a procedure called "Venus".

According to Dr. Randy Nordyke, who specializes in reducing cellulite for his clients and is owner and medical director of a medical spa in California, the radio frequency treatment called "Venus" is currently the most popular non-surgical cellulite treatment. It's a costly treatment – a series of 6 treatments will cost a patient about $2500 (the machine itself is about $90,000).

Dr. Nordyke recently made a statement that a brand new topical product, *NeriumFirm* http://aginginreverse.nerium.com/results/nerium-firm, first available in late April 2014, has shown as good (or better) results in as few as 3 weeks as the "Venus" treatments, and at a significantly lower price of $98!

After Rapid Weight Loss

During pregnancy, skin has the natural ability to stretch far beyond its original size and shape. It also has the natural ability to return back to normal within a fairly short time, especially during our 20's and early 30's.

Skin loses some of its elasticity with aging, so rapid weight loss can leave a lot of loose skin. Sometimes when people have lost a lot of weight due to fad dieting or weight-loss surgery they have resorted to surgery to remove large amounts of saggy, hanging skin.

Recent advances in skin firming creams are now helping people conquer extreme cases of loose skin non-surgically. Very dramatic results are being reported by people using *NeriumFirm* for 8 to 12 weeks in order to avoid more surgery after having undergone weight loss surgery.
http://aginginreverse.nerium.com/results/nerium-firm

Specialty Treatments

It's great to want to care for your skin in the most natural way possible. It can be a supportive, relaxing and fun treat, to make an appointment for a special facial treatment. This can be as simple and basic as a face massage, which is primarily about lymphatic drainage, and is wonderful for enhancing circulation and moving excess fluid, reducing puffiness and stress.

From time to time you may want to enhance your home skin care with a visit to an aesthetician or a med-spa for a rejuvenation treatment. Jeanette Wirz, a clinical aesthetician in Tennessee, recommends monthly to quarterly facials that include a glycolic (or other type) peel depending on your skin type.

Stress Reduction

Stress is one of the leading causes of *free radicals* that spur on the aging process. Even though all stress isn't bad, it still needs managing in order to stay healthy.

Stress comes in many shapes and sizes, from extreme to exciting to nagging little things that just add up. Think about that for just a minute and consider how all those things look on your face as you are experiencing them.

Big horrible things, happy things, and little nagging things all have their individual expressions that show on your face. Over time, those expressions become permanently embedded as muscles fall into patterns of tension, and aging skin loses the elasticity it needs to bounce back.

Now take a minute to consider what lies beyond the expressions – the feelings that create the expressions. OK, you're off the hook for now, because we aren't going there. That's the realm of the therapy of your choice, not skincare advice. But if you have real monsters in your closet and you're looking for a supplement or serum that will chase them away, let me assure you that your monsters aren't going to fall for that!

Now that we have that straight, there are lots of ways to ease the non-monster stress and lessen many of the lines and much of the dullness that might show on your face. If life offers you too many balls to juggle (or plates to spin, as some say), we need to find a way to stay calm.

Anything that gets you worked up, whether it's aggravating or super-exciting, can get your adrenalin rushing like Niagara Falls. Stress will make you forget to breathe, and you'll race around thinking a hand full of organic blue corn chips can suffice as a meal on your way out the door to your next "thing".

There are numerous ways to support your efforts to de-stress yourself, and many of them are free! We'll start with the free ones first. They're easier said than done, so lots of people just skip on to the things you have to pay for, but the free ones will help the most. I promise.

Breathe!

Let's start with breathing. It's imperative for maintaining life and it's supposed to be automatic, but it's astonishing how many adults routinely hold their breath. They do so without realizing it in response to life's stressors, from hunching over your computer all day, from driving for extended periods, or from just being too exhausted to stand up straight.

When you catch yourself in a mental state of anxiety or excitedly waiting for that last lottery number to match yours while holding your breath; stop and breathe. Holding your breath triggers the body's sympathetic nervous system response to impending danger, often known as the "fight or flight" response.

Here are some tips for reclaiming your breath. First, let's tame the "fight or flight" response that we don't need right now, because we're not running from bears or fighting our neighbors with spears anymore. If you feel out of sorts, have a panicky feeling, a headache, bellyache, backache, or become sleepless, take a second to stop. Stop whatever it is you're doing or thinking as soon as you realize it and **bring your focus to your breath**.

Focusing on the actual activity of breathing helps push other thoughts out of your mind. Even if it's only for a moment it puts you in contact with your body's inner "reset button". First, push out the old air you've been holding out of your lungs. As you do that, really focus solely on the activity of exhalation. Then let your next breath come in naturally and big, perhaps even a bit jaggedly as your muscles let go of their holding patterns. This allows your body to absorb oxygen to its deprived cells.

That first big breath will want to escape quickly so take advantage of it and turn it into a sigh of relief. This allows your body and especially your abdomen to relax for a moment before you inhale again. Really make it a convincing sigh of relief! Use it to let go of the tension in your jaw, forehead, neck, tummy, low back or wherever you're holding stress. Allow your mind to empty, setting aside all the jammed-up, busy, stressful thoughts and letting your whole body, and especially your face, soften a bit.

With the initial wave of tension cleared out, you can start taking more mindful deep breaths to nourish and calm your body, reminding it that all is well. With your next exhalation, another sigh of relief while relaxing your belly and emptying your mind. Let that stressed out feeling flow out with it, imagining it going deep into the ground, never to return.

Some stresses will be easier to push out than others. So whether it takes 3 breaths or 10 or more, be assured that you're doing the first best thing for managing stress by taking the time for intentional breathing. Deep breathing slows your adrenalin, calms your mind, and gives you an opportunity to shift your perspective away from whatever had you in knots.

Spend a few minutes before bedtime focused on intentional breathing and releasing all stressful thoughts. Releasing old patterns will go a long way toward helping you get a restorative night's sleep.

Sleep

Sleep is known as "the silent healer". It's called *beauty sleep* for a good reason! While you're getting a good night's sleep, your "inner physician" is very busy as your body repairs, rebalances and rejuvenates itself. The cellular renewal of our skin is fastest at night and effective night creams are formulated to support this process.

Lack of sleep seems to affect the skin more than it does other organs. Quality sleep promotes a decreased state of inflammation in the body. Levels of the stress hormones (adrenalin and cortisol) are at their lowest, and insulin production drops. Meanwhile growth hormone functions effectively 'wake up' and initiate cell repair during the Delta stage (the deepest sleep stage).

At the same time, "collagen production is accelerated, reducing evaporation and maximizing water retention in the epidermal/dermal junction, says Beverly Hills dermatologist Dr. Harold Lancer. Water retention within the skin is a key to fewer lines and smoother complexion.

Poor sleep can greatly interfere with this restorative cycle and lead to a dull, dehydrated appearance, as well as, skin sensitivity and irritation due to a reduction in protective capabilities.

Experts suggest 7 to 9 hours of sleep per night. Seven seems to be the minimum for giving your skin the time it needs to get through its entire restorative process. Eight is optimum, and enough for most adults. Sleeping much longer than that can have us waking up looking as puffy and feeling as sluggish as if we had slept only 3 hours.

The old adage, "an hour of sleep before midnight is worth three afterwards" does have truth behind it. A recent article from doctoroz.com explains that the deepest and most regenerative sleep occurs between 10pm and 2am.

More tried and true recommendations for maximizing your beauty sleep include:

- Sleep on your back (with a pillow under your knees). Stomach sleeping presses creases into your face that become permanent over time, and side sleeping can create accordion pleats across your chest.

- Try to stick to a regular bedtime and waking schedule, even on the weekends.

- Be sure your bedroom is dark. If your alarm clock is lighted make sure it's red. Red light does not disturb sleep, but other light colors do. Cover up any light from smoke alarms or other "always on" devices that might be in the bedroom. Lights and energy from computers and WiFi equipment can be very sleep disruptive, so locate them in another room in the house.

- Avoid caffeinated beverages long before bedtime.

- Get some kind of exercise during the day, but not immediately before going to bed.

- Refer to the focused breathing discussed earlier. It will calm your nervous system to help you relax quickly and sleep better.

Exercise and Massage

Exercise brings a boost in tension-relieving brain chemicals like dopamine, serotonin, and norepinephrine, which can lower stress levels and diminish the effects of aging. Yoga is particularly helpful for reducing the level of stress hormones, so consider incorporating it into your exercise plan to support clear, radiant skin.

The National Sleep Foundation has reported that exercising in the afternoon helps promote better sleep and cuts the time it takes to drift off into your beauty sleep. Sometimes planned exercise, or other physical exertion like yard work or carrying a bunch of heavy groceries for awhile, can cause soreness and muscle fatigue. Let go of the tension buildup by relaxing in a bath with 1 to 2 cups of Epsom salt. This can offer great relief to aching muscles and help to balance fluid in your skin.

Massage and other bodywork modalities such as lymphatic drainage therapy (LDT) or craniosacral therapy can help increase circulation in the skin. These techniques help to move excess fluid out, while supporting the de-stressing process for body, mind and spirit.

Mind & Spirit

"To be beautiful means to be yourself. You don't need to be accepted by others. You need to accept yourself." ~Thich Nhat Hanh

Our thoughts and emotions can have an impact on not only how we perceive our skin from our mirror reflection, but on the actual condition of our skin. So reducing mental stress can go a long way to keeping your skin healthy.

According to Dr. Derek H. Jones, a Los Angeles based dermatologist, there seems to be a relationship between the mind and the skin. Although he says proving this scientifically is difficult, he says, "It is well known that when someone has psoriasis, stress tends to make the problem worse ... stress really does alter the immune system".

Audry Kunin, MD from Kansas City says, "It is so common for my patients to report when they leave town on some relaxing vacation, their psoriasis or eczema almost magically resolves."

Ted A. Grossbart, PhD, a Harvard Medical School psychologist, says, "Our bodies respond to an imagined situation as if it were real. If you picture yourself sitting by the fire, your toes actually get warmer."

Beauty is self-defined and self-created. Sure, it's influenced by all the artificial images that are promoted to us as beauty. However, absolute acceptance of who you are and what you have to offer will allow you to present the most beautiful YOU. Scrutinizing, analyzing, and criticizing every little line, bump and freckle keeps you uncomfortable in your skin and sends negative messages to your cells. Make a commitment to yourself to catch the negative, self-critical thoughts and begin reprogramming them to look for the positive aspects in yourself and in others.

Embracing the suggestions, "don't sweat the small stuff", "roll with the punches", "go with the flow" can go a long way to reducing the lines on your face. Carrying "an attitude of gratitude" shifts your mind into positive high gear and softens your expression, helping to keep frown lines from forming. Try joining the "happiness movement" and seeking joy in all you do!

When you feel naturally joyous, it shows on your face and gives you more energy to support your entire well-being. Keeping a personal connection to the Higher Power that guides your spirit through life, whether you call it God, or some other name, helps keep you on a positive path when other people and events around you may try to pull you down.

Connecting and sharing time with friends and family, meeting new like-minded people through activities you enjoy, and creating a positive network helps feed your spirit. The first time you consciously "pay it forward" in some way, notice the gleeful sparkle you feel. If there's a mirror nearby, you will see it in your eyes. Know that it's dancing in every cell of your body and your skin is part of that dance.

Looking Younger: Nourish Your Skin From The Inside Out

Hydrate

Drink the cleanest water you can access. Every system in your body relies on water. Dehydration really shows up on your skin, and contributes to decreased brain function and fatigue as well.

Space your water intake throughout the day, instead of chugging down a liter bottle after lunch. This will allow your body to utilize and distribute the water in a more efficient way to nourish your cells and ease the process of waste removal.

According to the Institute of Medicine, an adequate daily fluid intake for men is 3 liters, and 2.2 liters for women. Ideally, about 20% of your hydration should come from fresh fruits and vegetables, which are naturally high in water content (see the nutrition section below).

So the conventional wisdom to drink eight 8-ounce glasses of water per day still holds true. Many liquids consumed may count toward your total. However, making water your beverage of choice keeps you from adding extra calories!

A recommendation from the Mayo clinic is to consider other factors that require extra hydration. Vigorous exercise, a hot climate, breastfeeding, an illnesses with fever, vomiting, or diarrhea all place a higher demand on the water resources of your body.

Nourish

The best "diet" is eating REAL food! Your best choices include:

* Fresh seasonal vegetables
* Fresh fruits
* Brown rice
* Quinoa
* Wild-caught fish
* Clean meats like 100% grass-fed beef, or pasture-raised, organic chicken or turkey

Choose organic foods whenever possible. While foods labeled "all natural" have the possibility of being ok, the term "natural" (which has no real legal nutrition definition) is often used in misleading packaging. Learning to read and understand food labeling is important when seeking healthier choices for yourself and your family.

Tip: For more information on reading food labels successfully, see page 98 of *Beating Sugar Addiction For Dummies* (BeatingSugarAddiction.com).

In some people, certain foods may create an allergic or intolerance response that may show up in their skin condition as itching, rashes, or other types of eruptions.

For example, Lisa found that when she eliminated gluten from her diet, her severe acne cleared up completely within a few months. She had not been diagnosed with celiac disease, but gluten was a factor that compromised her overall health enough to show up on her skin.

Informative gluten-free resources include *Wheat Belly: Lose the Wheat, Lose the Weight* and *Find Your Path Back To Health* by William Davis, MD. I also recommend GlutenDude.com.

Understanding Free Radicals and Antioxidants

Free radicals

Free radicals are unstable molecules that are quick to react with other compounds, including your cells. A free radical in your body can be the equivalent of a political extremist looking for co-conspirators. Free radical *oxidation* is part of normal bodily function and metabolism, but when there are too many free radicals, it can lead to cell damage, inflammation, and disease. This shows on your body as premature aging, wrinkles, tissue deterioration, and other internal diseases.

Keeping free radicals in check is why we hear so much about the value of antioxidants!

Some of the big contributing factors to an over abundance of free radicals in the body are:
  * Processed foods
  * Stress
  * Smoke (any kind)
  * Pesticides
  * Environmental toxins
  * Drugs (prescribed or recreational)
  * UV rays
  * Radiation
  * Rancid oils in food and lotions

Processed, packaged foods contain numerous chemical preservatives, sugars, and hydrogenated oils that contribute to an overabundance of free radicals in our bodies.

Antioxidants

The best way to support your body's chemistry lab is to choose foods that help balance these chemical reactions. You want a healthy functioning body that doesn't have a tendency toward diseased processes. Certain foods supply elements that stay stable even as they give away an electron to stabilize a free radical. These elements are called antioxidants.

One of the easiest ways to find antioxidant rich foods is to look at the color. Brightly colored foods tend to indicate a high antioxidant value. A darker color = more antioxidants.

Good examples are:

Bananas
Blueberries
Broccoli
Carrots
Kale
Nuts (also contain healthy essential fats)
Red beans
Red or purple grapes
Spinach
Strawberries
Wild salmon

Major antioxidants include vitamins A, C, and E; coenzyme Q10, and *anthocyanins*. Anthocyanins protect cells from damage and heal already damaged cells. They're found in foods with purple skins. Isothiocynates are important for detoxification and are found in broccoli, spinach and parsley. Other antioxidants are flavonoids, lutein, lycopene, and selenium.

Essential Fatty Acids

Essential fatty acids are polyunsaturated fats that are essential for proper development and functioning of the human body. Essential fats are crucial for the formation of healthy cell membranes.

Our bodies do not produce these specific fats, so they must be obtained through our foods. The main essential fatty acids are Omega-3 and Omega-6, and are found in a wide variety of foods. A balanced ratio of Omega-6 to Omega-3 ranges from 1:1 to 4:1. However, the typical Western diet is extremely unbalanced and ends up more like 10:1 to as much as 25:1.

Many foods contain far more Omega-6 than we really need. So one of the keys for supporting optimal health and skin condition is choosing foods every day that supply more Omega-3.

The very best food sources for Omega-3, according to The George Mateljan Foundation in the book "The World's Healthiest Foods" are flax seeds, walnuts, sardines, and wild salmon.
Other good sources include soybeans, chia seeds, dark green vegetables like collards and kale, and brussel sprouts.

There are many healthy benefits to consuming foods that contain plenty of essential fatty acids. This includes the regulation of proper thyroid and adrenal activity, as well as, the development and function of the brain and nervous system.

Omega-3 fats possess natural anti-inflammatory qualities that help to regulate blood pressure and support healthy skin. A diet low in omega-3 fats may contribute to skin problems such as dryness, eczema, or dandruff as well as brittle hair and splitting nails.

Anti-inflammatory Foods

Processed foods, environmental factors and certain lifestyle choices can lead to a state of inflammation in the body. Chronic inflammation brings a host of health compromising conditions that include a variety of skin conditions like those mentioned above.

Many foods are famous for their anti-inflammatory properties – and all of them are fresh, not processed foods. It seems like a no-brainer, but in our fast-paced lives these days, packaged stuff is easy and relatively cheap.

So instead of rushing out the door with a pop-tart, stock up on bananas and organic apples which are equally portable but much more nourishing. And for some protein and healthy fat to accompany your worthy carbohydrates, look for the super portable/packable nut butters from Justin's. Many grocery stores and health food stores are carrying these. I found them at my local Kroger store, in the 'healthy' section. Visit Justins.com.

When you aren't in a rush, enjoy creating a new relationship with foods that really nourish your personal "chemistry lab" and see the results on your skin and in your eyes when you look in the mirror.

Invest in a great book like *The World's Healthiest Foods* by George Mateljan, and keep it in your kitchen. That way, when you explore a piece of produce or other fresh food you've never tried before (like Swiss chard, beet greens, dandelion greens, or eggplant) you can quickly find information. Mateljan's book gives you tips on the best way to prepare the foods and store it, along with nutritional information and recipes. Common foods you're more familiar with are in there too.

Dr. Andrew Weil posts an anti-inflammatory food pyramid on his website, which you can easily access at

http://www.drweil.com/drw/u/ART02995/Dr-Weil-Anti-Inflammatory-Food-Pyramid.html.

At last, fruits and vegetables have taken the largest seat at the base of the pyramid! Dr. Weil's second tier includes whole and cracked grains, beans and legumes, and an occasional dose of pasta. In the middle section of this pyramid we find healthy fats, with a suggested 5 to 7 servings daily.

While this is more servings per day than any other food group, a serving of healthy fat should be drastically smaller than a serving of any other food. If you visit the website and click on the tier, you get a window with more information about serving size. A serving of healthy fat is very small. For example, 1 teaspoon (not Tablespoon) of extra-virgin olive oil; 2 walnuts; 1 Tablespoon of flaxseed; 1 ounce of avocado.

The middle third of this pyramid includes protein sources like fish and seafood, whole soy foods, cooked Asian mushrooms, lean meats, natural cheeses, omega-3 enriched eggs, and yogurt. The upper third allows for an unlimited amount of healthy herbs and spices like garlic, turmeric, cinnamon and ginger, 2-4 cups of white or green tea per day, nutritional supplements as needed, an option for red wine, and at the pinnacle of the pyramid... plain dark chocolate (sparingly, of course, and the darker the better).

Essential Vitamins and Minerals For Ageless Skin

Most of your vitamin and mineral support should come from eating healthy food. However, supplementation is often helpful or necessary to support optimum health and function.

Key vitamins and minerals for healthiest skin condition include:

Vitamin A - necessary for healing and construction of new skin tissue. Vitamin A is a fat-soluble vitamin, which is significant for a couple of reasons. First, the fat-soluble vitamins (A, D, E and K) are less likely to be lost when food is cooked.

Fat-soluble vitamins are stored by the body within the liver and fatty tissues. Because of this, most people do not need a lot of supplementation of these vitamins when a healthy diet is maintained.

The 10 best food sources for vitamin A are:

Bell peppers
Calf's liver
Carrots
Collard greens
Kale
Parsley
Romaine lettuce
Spinach
Sweet potatoes
Swiss chard

Other good sources of vitamin A include cantaloupe, winter squash, apricots, broccoli and tomatoes.

B vitamins - B vitamins are usually grouped in supplements as **B complex** because they work together as a team. In general, they seem to work best when they're received in a balanced way. They are water soluble (as is Vitamin C), which means they're not stored in the body and must be replenished every day.

Since they're often found together in a variety of foods, they were originally thought to be only one vitamin. As scientific research and development improved, each of the B vitamins revealed a distinct molecular structure.

The process of discovery and naming of the B group resulted in some confusion. B4, B8, B10, B11 and a host of other elements were eliminated. While they might be interesting and useful they are not considered vitamins. With the numbering confusion, it's becoming more common to see them referred to by name.

All eight of the B vitamins are referenced by individual names and numbers:

* Thiamin is Vitamin B_1
* Riboflavin is Vitamin B_2
* Niacin or Niacinamide is Vitamin B_3
* Pantothenic acid is Vitamin B_5
* Pyridoxine is Vitamin B_6
* Biotin is Vitamin B_7
* Folate (or folic acid) is Vitamin B_9
* Cobalamin is Vitamin B_{12} (supplemental form is usually cyanocobalamin or the more effective form, methylcobalamin)

B vitamins play important roles in cell metabolism and are easily depleted in stressful conditions that place high demands on your adrenal glands, brain function and/or muscular system. And, since stress is one of the major factors in free radical production which contributes to aging skin the Bs are high on our list! Your multi-vitamin/mineral supplement should have a B-complex built in.

The B vitamins are plentiful in whole foods, so eating a variety of fresh vegetable, fruits and whole grains will supply most of the B vitamins you need. Animal foods are the only natural sources of Vitamin B_{12} so if you choose a vegan diet, B_{12} supplementation is essential for optimum health.

Vitamin C - fights free radicals and strengthens the capillaries that feed the skin. It also supports wound healing and is necessary for the formation of collagen, which gives skin its flexibility. The best sources for Vitamin C are very fresh vegetables and fruits.

You don't have to limit yourself to just oranges for vitamin C. Papaya, raw broccoli, and fresh bell peppers offer up more Vitamin C per serving than citrus fruits. Vitamin C is highly sensitive to air, water, and temperature, so cooking vegetables and fruits can result in the loss of 30% or more of the vitamin C content.

Vitamin E - Helps protect skin from ultraviolet light and protects against free radicals that can damage skin cells and contribute to aging. Top food sources for Vitamin E are sunflower seeds, swiss chard, almonds, and spinach. Cold pressed oils like olive oil and sunflower seed oil are also high in vitamin E.

Selenium – Is a mineral that acts as an antioxidant in tandem with vitamin E for protection against free radical damage. Only tiny amounts of selenium are needed every day. A discoloration of hair or skin can indicate a need for more selenium. Excellent food sources of selenium include cod, tuna, salmon, cremini and shiitake mushrooms, turkey, lamb, oats, and brown rice.

Zinc - This essential mineral is required for collagen formation. It helps promote wound healing, and may help prevent acne and regulate the activity of oil glands. Some of the best food sources for zinc include pumpkin seeds, spinach, grass-fed beef, and calf's liver.

Copper - works in balance with zinc and Vitamin C to form elastin and collagen in the skin. Copper is found in many of the same foods as zinc, as well as in copper plumbing and some cookware.

CoQ10 - (CoEnzyme Q10, also known as ubiquinone) is a fat soluble, vitamin-like antioxidant that's produced naturally within the human body and is found in every cell and tissue. It's a key component in the essential production of energy for every cell in the body, and is instrumental in neutralizing free radicals and keeping skin healthy.

CoQ10 helps protect the deeper layers of skin from damage caused by UVA light, which can show up as loss of elasticity leading to wrinkles, sagging skin, hyperpigmentation or even some cancerous lesions. The level of natural CoQ10 within the skin is fairly low in childhood and rises to a peak level between ages 20 - 30, then gradually decreases with age.

In the anti-aging realm, there is probably more interest in and talk about the uses and benefits of CoQ10 than another other supplement. So, you will hear about it again in the next section as we discuss supporting your skin from the outside in.

This list of supportive supplements could go on and on since optimum general health equals optimum skin health. Remember the more you strive to eat with the understanding that food is your best medicine, the more you support your wellness and youthful appearance from the inside out.

Most of us live busy, active, hectic and stressful lives and don't always manage to eat the way we should. Many people wisely add vitamin and mineral supplements to fill in the blanks, so to speak. What most people don't realize is that a poor quality supplement does them little or no good. The low-quality brands that are available off the shelves in drugstores and discount chains are generally made from cheap ingredients and poorly absorbed forms of minerals. A high-quality supplement will

1) Test well in the lab for purity and labeling accuracy (look for the GMP stamp, which stands for Good Manufacturing Practices certification), and
2) Contain high-quality, bioavailable forms of nutrients.

I suggest the **Science Line Nutrition** multi-vitamin for my clients, available at GettingFit.com/shop.

Skincare Ingredients – What You Do and Don't Want To Find There

Understanding Alcohols in Skincare Products

The term "alcohol" may easily be misunderstood, especially with regard to what's in personal care products. There are two general types of alcohols you may find on product labels:

1) The kind you really don't want to find in your skin products is the drying type, which may be listed as 'ethanol', 'SD alcohol', 'denatured alcohol', methanol, benzyl alcohol, isopropyl alcohol.

2) The other type of alcohol you will commonly see is a group of waxy, moisturizing fatty alcohols derived from natural oils and fats. They are used as emulsifiers or thickeners in lotions and creams. These may be listed as 'cetearyl alcohol', 'stearyl alcohol', or 'cetyl alcohol'.

Key Ingredients

Leading skincare products all tend to use some similar ingredients as the background mix for proper blending and appealing texture. The "key" ingredients do vary, and here is a list of 10 key ingredients that you will be happy to find in your skincare products:

- **Hyaluronic acid** - (may be listed as Sodium hyaluronate) - the most powerful and natural moisturizer and humectant (moisture attractor), this is a naturally occuring substance with our skin and other tissues, which declines with age. Topical use can help smooth and soften skin, reducing the appearance of wrinkles.

- **Glycosaminoglycans** - the body's natural moisturizers, helping to attract water into skin and keep it hydrated. (Hyaluronic acid is part of this group.) When added to skincare products, these deeply penetrating molecules can help hydrate, repair and revitalize your skin.

- **Aloe barbadensis** - has a long history of healing and anti-inflammatory properties. Helps moisturize and protect skin, stimulates cells that produce collagen, protects from UV rays.

- **Biotech proprietary blends** - game-changing biotech ingredients like the patented extract in *Nerium AD* products (known as NAE-8, a nature-based and science-developed melding Aloe Barbadensis leaf juice and Nerium Oleander extract). This was an accidental discovery which has shown unprecedented results as a non-prescription multi-purpose anti-aging ingredient that works! The Nerium Oleander extract has proven to condition, smooth, and enhance the radiance of the skin, as well as to reduce the appearance of fine lines, wrinkles, discoloration, enlarged pores, uneven texture, and aging skin – all with just one product!

- **Ubiquinone** (CoQ10) - a powerful antioxidant that has been shown to support when applied to the skin's surface as well as when taken internally.

- **Vitamins: Vitamin C** (various forms of ascorbate/ascorbyl/ascorbic) - a powerful antioxidant that helps increase collagen production in skin and helps combat sun damage.

- **Vitamin E** (Alpha-tocopherol or Tocopheryl acetate) - provides antioxidant properties and some photoprotection by absorbing the energy from UV exposure.

- **Vitamin A** - One of the most well-known anti-aging ingredients is retinol (the strongest non-prescription form of Vitamin A with a common side-effect of skin irritation), and its gentler form, retinyl palmitate.

- **Camellia Sinensis or Camellia Oleifera** (green or white tea leaf extract) - a plant extract with well documented antioxidant and anti-inflammatory properties.

- **Niacinamide** - a derivative of vitamin-B3, it has been shown to reduce the appearance of dark discolorations and may also help reduce inflammation.

- **Peptides** - may be listed as "proprietary peptide matrix" or "proprietary protein", these amino acids (the building blocks of protein) function as moisture-binding agents that help promote the natural production of collagen and elastin fibers

- **Alpha-hydroxy acids** - the most commonly used alpha-hydroxy acid is glycolic acid (derived from sugar cane), but you may also see lactic acid (derived from sour milk), malic acid (derived from apples), citric acid (from citrus fruits), or tartaric acid (from grape wine). These help encourage exfoliation, and enhance the cell turnover rate, as well as collagen production

Ingredient "Watch" List

Sometimes what's **NOT** in product is just as important to look for as what IS in it! There are many ingredients in skin care products. From shampoos and rinses all the way to high-end moisturizers and specialty treatments that are known to do more harm than good. Choosing healthy skin care products requires diligent label-reading, just like making healthy food choices.

Here are some ingredients that should make you want to put the bottle back on the shelf because you don't want them in your skincare products:

* **Triclosan**: This is an antimocrobial chemical and might be found in antibacterial soaps and deodorants, and possibly even in toothpaste. Triclosan is a known skin irritant and a disruptor to the endocrine system, most particularly the thyroid and reproductive hormones. Studies are also showing that it may contribute to causing certain bacteria to become antibiotic-resistant.

* **Mineral oil / petrolatum** - while there are a few instances where a petroleum-based product may be useful or even preferable, anti-aging face products are

much more suited to plant-based oils. Petroleum products are considered to be 'comedogenic', which means they are likely to clog pores, leading to blackheads and whiteheads. And by all means, avoid chapped lip products that contain mineral oil or petrolatum - these actually promote chapping! Petroleum products sit on the surface of skin, creating a barrier, rather than providing a vehicle for the nourishing ingredients of a skincare product to penetrate into the deeper layers. They promote photosensitivity, dry skin and chapping by interfering with the body's own natural moisturizing mechanism. Look for gentler, more nourishing moisturizers like beeswax, shea butter, or castor oil.

* **Parabens** - these are ingredients that are often used to inhibit microbial growth and extend the shelf-life of a product. They are known to be toxic and frequently cause allergic reactions and skin rashes.

* **Synthetic colors**: FD&C colors (indicated on labels by D&C or FD&C, followed by a number) are derived from coal tar or petroleum and are skin irritants as well as suspected carcinogens and a possible contributor to ADHD in children.

* **Synthetic fragrance**: also known as "**fragrance**", refers to a mysterious and proprietary concoction of chemicals to create a particular artificial smell. Synthetic fragrances in skin care products, perfumes, and laundry products are among the leading causes of skin irritation and allergies.

* **Gluten**: With the huge increase in awareness of gluten sensitivity or complete intolerance (due to celiac

disease), avoiding gluten on the skin can be as important as avoiding it in foods. A benefit to avoiding this ingredient means that most likely the product was formulated without a lot of other bad stuff as well.

Sun Damage

Choosing skincare products containing the "good guy" ingredients discussed above, while avoiding the "bad guy" ingredients will go a long way toward keeping your skin nourished and moisturized from the outside. Your next responsibility is to avoid damaging your skin from the outside – literally. Excessive outdoor sun exposure will wreck your skin faster than any parabens or synthetic fragrances.

Wearing a hat can help shade your face and protect your scalp when outdoors. Specially designed UPF (ultraviolet protection factor) clothing like the great designs from companies like Columbia, Coolibar, and others can provide added protection from sun and wind damage.

Exposure Management

When I was born, the pediatrician advised my mother to be sure I was exposed to 15 minutes of sunlight every day. So, I spent my early days in diapers on Waikiki beach. Tough life, I know. But 15 minutes is just a tease!

Pre-teen summers at the lake gave way to college sunbathing on the dorm roof slathered in a home-brew of baby oil and iodine, along with a part-time job as a lifeguard at the community pool. I never got a severe sunburn, and I wonder if it was because my Mom heeded the doctor's advice when I was a baby. My sister was born 3 1/2 years later in the midst of Minnesota winter, and she has the fairest skin ever, loaded with freckles and a history of sunburns. I'd love to see some scientific research noting these patterns.

Just as plants need sunlight to manufacture their essential chlorophyl, we need sunlight to naturally manufacture our essential Vitamin D, dubbed "the sunshine vitamin". Vitamin D is necessary for healthy immune system function, calcium absorption, bone health and more.

There are very few food sources for Vitamin D, primarily oily fish such as salmon and cod liver oil, and egg yolks. Our bodies naturally produce Vitamin D when we are exposed to sunlight without sunscreen.

The sun has been made our aging and skin cancer enemy, and consequently most of us are now deficient in Vitamin D. So now doctors prescribe high doses of Vitamin D and full coverage sunscreen instead of sensible exposure to sunlight, while scientists argue that getting a little sunshine on your skin helps reduce the incidence of other types of cancer such as colon, breast, and kidney. For sporting an ageless look, tanning beds are not your friend! Enough said.

Sun Management

Accepting that our beloved sunlight does carry dangers with over exposure, what is reasonable? As with most anything in life, self-respect and moderation are key. Understanding your innate skin coloring can also guide you. Very fair, easily freckled people need to take far more precaution than someone with dark skin in order to avoid sun damage.

Protect yourself from the aging and damaging effects of ultraviolet light from the sun by avoiding direct sun exposure during the hours between 10:00am and 4:00pm. This is when the suns rays are most potent. An easy rule of thumb is to remember that if your shadow is shorter than you are, the sun is still too harsh to be in for long. "Short shadow, seek shade!"

Any time you're going to be in direct sun for more than a total of 15-20 minutes a day, you must cover up if you want to keep your skin looking ageless.

A wide-brimmed hat, sunglasses, and tightly woven fabrics (darker colors are best) are effective at blocking much of the damaging rays. There are clothing lines that specialize in using fabrics that provide a high level of ultraviolet protection factor (see the "Protection" section above). For skin areas that are not covered by clothing, and for extra protection on the face, sunscreen or sunblock is always recommended by dermatologists.

Sun Protection

Make your sun protection an additional step to your skin care routine. Allow your moisturizer a few minutes to absorb into your skin before applying a sun protection product with SPF ranging between 15 - 50, depending on your natural skin coloring and how long you may be in the sun.

UVB rays are more intense during the summer months, but UVA rays are pretty much the same all year, so if you're going out to shovel snow for an hour, don't forget to protect your face!

Sunscreen or Sunblock?

In chemical sunscreens, the active ingredients act as filters to reduce the penetration of ultraviolet radiation into the skin. Avobenzone and Mexoryl SX are chemical sunscreens that provide protection from UVA rays.

Some people are sensitive to chemical sunscreens and fare better with sunblocks.

Just because you've applied sunscreen, don't forget to incorporate the other protection factors like seeking shade, avoiding peak hours and wearing protective clothing. Sunscreens break down once absorbed into the skin and lose their effectiveness within a fairly short time. Let the SPF number guide you to the amount of protection, not the length of time you can safely stay in the sun. Many reports cite an increase in severe sunburns in people using sunscreen because they fail to reapply it.

Sunblock products physically block both UVA and UVB light, primarily with the use of zinc oxide and/or titanium dioxide as the active ingredients. Mineral-based sunblocks are preferable for anyone with sensitive skin, and for those less likely to reapply during their sun exposure time.

Some products combine both sunscreen chemicals and sun-blocking minerals. Whether you choose a chemical sunscreen, a sunblock, or a blend you need to be sure to use "broad spectrum" product, meaning that it protects from both UVA and UVB types of rays.

My personal favorite is Blue Lizard "Sensitive", with the active ingredients zinc oxide and titanium dioxide, because it doesn't contain any chemical sunscreens, fragrance, or parabens. "Sensitive" is SPF 30+, Broad Spectrum UVA/UVB protection, and after a few minutes it's not as pasty white as many of the others I've tried.

For the safest and most effective results, please educate yourself and choose your sun protection carefully. Don't succumb to marketing campaigns or just reach for the cheapest, or most familiar name, or one that smells nice. A super-high SPF number (above 50) is often misleading marketing, and some sunscreens contain chemicals that can do more harm than good. Also, avoid spray-on sunscreens. Even though they seem like a convenient and easy plan, aside from the inhalation risks it's too easy to miss some spots or apply too little.

The Environmental Working Group (EWG) has an extensive listing of sun protection products and an approval rating system for each. This is a fantastic reference for further educating yourself and choosing a good product: http://www.ewg.org/2014sunscreen

More label-reading for you! Some ingredients to avoid in your sunscreen include:

Vitamin A (also known as retinyl palmitate or retinol): While Vitamin A and its derivatives are supportive as an anti-aging ingredient when used at night, with exposure to sunlight they degrade quickly and go from being supportive to being damaging. Retinols were found in about 20% of the beach and sport sunscreens examined by EWG.

Oxybenzone: There is evidence that this ingredient (which soaks through skin) can trigger allergic skin reactions in sensitive individuals, and may cause hormone disruption by acting as an estrogen in the body. Oxybenzone was found in nearly 50% of the sunscreens examined by EWG in 2014!

Anti-aging Products

Even people in their 20's are becoming concerned about signs of aging skin, which to someone in their 50's may sound funny, but I hear it often. And, it isn't just women who are concerned with keeping their appearance youthful. We live in a very image-conscious society where "putting your best face forward" goes a long way towards helping both men and women achieve their personal and business goals. Not to mention the self-confidence that comes with feeling good about the reflection you see in the mirror every morning!

The good news is that you have hundreds and maybe thousands of choices when it comes to anti-aging products. The bad news is, you have hundreds and maybe thousands of choices when it comes to anti-aging products.

Have you ever noticed that the beauty counter is the first, and largest, section you see when you enter the front of a major department store? How in the world do you make the right choice(s)? Do I really need the 7-step product line? Or would the 5-step product line be better? Could I get the same results with that 3-step system? Is there any way that I could get great results just using one product instead of some complicated process?

Nerium International has created NeriumAD Age-Defying treatment, a night cream that addresses the appearance of multiple concerns (fine lines and wrinkles, discoloration, uneven skin texture and aging skin) with just one product. The results from their 28-day clinical trials, using advanced facial scanning technology (originally designed for detecting scratches on microchips), revealed a remarkable average of 30% improvement in deep lines, fine lines and even the emerging lines we don't see yet.

For more information visit Aginginreverse.nerium.com/results.

Recommendations from friends can be the best way to find a great product. Notice your friends who routinely look great and ask those friends what skincare product(s) they're using. Look at the labels though!

Some of the best products aren't even available in the department stores or drug stores. Many of us have friends who have chosen to partner with relationship marketing companies because of outstanding products and an entrepreneurial business opportunity. Don't be afraid to be supportive of your friend's business, especially if you can tell they are using something that really works for them.

Often times (but not always) these types of products have unique ingredients and formulas that you won't find in any of the department store products. Additionally, unlike department stores, most products sold through your friends' businesses will come with a 30-day money back guarantee so you can see if it is a good product for you - risk free!

How To Phase In New Products

When trying a new product, only use the new product - don't mix with your old products.

Every time a new product is introduced to your daily routine, it is possible that you may encounter a temporary reaction. Your skin must become accustomed to a product to determine how it interacts with your skin long-term.

Also, to help avoid irritation, it's best to use a sunscreen that's separate from your specialized skincare treatment product. When using a daytime moisturizer, allow it several minutes to absorb into your skin before applying your sunscreen.

If you experience minor irritations, give yourself time to adjust to using a new product. You might try using less of the product at one time or using every other day during the first week or so. If you have minor to mild irritation, it's recommended that you allow at least two to three weeks for your skin to acclimate. If you have a severe reaction, you should stop using any new products and seek medical advice.

If you do choose to use multiple products, you may want to test a small area with both products to see if there is any reaction to the combination. Whenever applying multiple products, use the following rules: apply clearest first, moving then to most opaque, and apply thinnest first then to thickest.

Since you look at yourself in the mirror every day and subtle changes may go unnoticed, it is a good idea to track your results. So before you start with a new product experience, take a series of "before" photos with your cell phone camera. Be sure to take front, both sides, and zero in on any problem areas.

After 3-4 weeks, take the exact same "after" photos. Digital cameras are very revealing. When the photos are enlarged it's easy to determine if wrinkles and pores are getting smaller, if skin tone and texture have improved, if skin is tightening, if discoloration is diminishing, etc.

It's important to understand that there's not one product on the market that works for every single person. So look for products that have a 30-day "money back guarantee". If you buy a new product and seem to have a sensitivity or a reaction to it, there are a few things to consider:

* Did you use another product under or over it? Sometimes different ingredient blends don't play well together.

* Did you accidentally leave traces of soap or cleanser on your skin before applying the anti-aging product?

* Are you taking a medication that may be causing a photosensitive response to sunlight?
If there doesn't seem to be any other contributing factor take time to observe. What is the reaction like?

If it's a minor breakout, slight sensation of tingling or tightness, or a little bit of an exacerbation of what you have already been experiencing and want to resolve, give it a few days and see if things calm down. It's not uncommon for skin to go through an "adjustment" phase with a more effective new product. There can be a clearing effect before the really nice changes start. Sometimes it may be helpful to use a new product every other day at first.

If there is more than just a superficial reaction and involves hives, headache, sneezing then you are most likely having an allergic response to something in the product and should not continue using it. Return it and get your money back so you can explore a different product.

Sometimes people ask me if they will have to use an anti-aging product "forever" to keep the results. The answer is ... yes ... skin may seem constant, but it is ever-changing. True, it continually renews itself. Also true, the aging process does not stop.

Your skin is your companion for life, so making a commitment to care for it well, and forever, is an excellent choice! When you find a great product or products that work well and give the results you're seeking, then enjoy that investment in yourself. And, with new biotech breakthrough products like NeriumAD, people are enjoying truly remarkable results over time, without using invasive options like fillers, botox, lasers or surgery.

For more information visit:
Aginginreverse.theneriumlook.com.

Cosmetic Dos and Don'ts

Are you confused with all the choices and rules, rules, rules? Page after page in beauty blogs, magazines, and Youtube videos tell you Do This, Don't Do That, and Buy My Stuff. This section will give you some important but simple principles for you to apply when choosing cosmetics.

One of the most important factors in looking your best at any age, no matter your gender, is choosing to surround yourself in the right colors for your skin tone, which is often the biggest challenge. Knowing whether your personal palette is Winter, Summer, Spring or Autumn and what that means with regard to your best colors, can help you make better choices in your clothing and accessories as well as your makeup products.

In 1987 the best-selling author, Carole Jackson, gave us the guidance to choose our personal color palette based on the seasons in her book *Color Me Beautiful*. This was an enlightening and transformative book for me. It got me away from wearing clothes and makeup based on what was "in" according to the trends and wearing colors that suited my coloring instead. The difference was amazing! I started hearing things like, "you look great today" or "wow, your eyes are gorgeous" instead of "do you feel ok?" or "you look kind of tired today".

The Dos

Here are some guidelines for looking naturally great any time:

* For daytime when you want to look daytime-natural (only better) a "less is more" approach is mandatory. You can be ready in 5 minutes or less! Aging skin can actually look much older when too much makeup is applied.

* Use a lightweight moisturizer on your clean face followed by sunscreen (or use one of the approved moisturizer/sunscreen combinations from the list at: http://www.ewg.org/2014sunscreen/best-sunscreens/best-moisturizers-with-spf/

* The only must-have makeup item is something for lips! A little of the right color on your lips and/or a little gloss can do more to brighten up your face than anything else. It does need to be the right color! (refer to the info on colors, above) For a perfect and lasting lip color, check out Julia's Lip Tint at: http://www.juliasliptint.com/

* For covering "flaws" (discolorations and blemishes), use a tiny dab of concealer that most closely matches your skin coloring on blemishes or discolorations. Let it sit for a moment before blending gently upwards and outwards.

* For a smoother look, you may want to follow with a lightweight foundation, taking care to blend it around under your jaw line, not onto your neck, but gently blended toward it. If you tend to be oily a little translucent powder in the "T" zone (forehead and nose)

will cut the shine without weighing you down or making you look too made-up.

* Take a moment to check on your eyebrows. If they've gotten a little unruly, give them a quick shape-up. If you have bare spots, fill in with matching pencil and blend well.

* Daytime-natural eyes will dazzle with a neatly applied coat of non-waterproof mascara. Water based mascara is easier to remove and kinder to your eyelashes than the waterproof type. Save the waterproof stuff for weddings, funerals, and waterfront vacations.

* Using a nice fluffy professional blush brush to apply a hint of softly colored blush to the highest part of your check. Be sure the color is in your personal palette and complements your lipstick color, and blend the edges so that it looks like a natural blush, with no distinct line.

* Don't forget your earrings!

* For transitioning into evening.... blot any oiliness with special blotter paper or a tissue before adding a little more blush. Then use a light dusting of translucent powder, another coat of mascara and a slightly brighter lip color. Add eyeliner and eye shadow for a more dramatic look if you wish. Hint: If you're out with the girls, let your eyes be the feature of emphasis and downplay your lip color. If you are out on a date, you may want to play up your lip color with a matching lip-liner and a touch of gloss over your color.

The Don'ts

A few things to keep in mind as you plan your cosmetic routine:

* Don't go to bed without cleansing makeup and daily grime from your face!

* Don't match eye shadow to your eyes or your outfit. This will just make you look clueless, unless you did it on purpose for a "throwback to 70's/80's" look. Instead, choose a shade of brown that creates a soft shadow to draw attention to the natural light in your eyes. Don't distract by calling attention to the color around your eyes.

* Don't use old, clumpy mascara! If your mascara is clumping, throw it out and open a new tube. Mascara should be replaced every 1 to 3 months.

* Don't overdo it with glittery or shiny make-up. A little bit of glitter can put the "party" in your evening look, but avoid it if your outfit already has the "bling" going on. And definitely don't use it for daytime. Instead choose foundations or light powders that boost luminosity or radiance to create a timeless look.

* Don't forget to check your expression! Are you carrying around any negative feelings that are reflecting in your eyes? Are you carrying tension around your mouth, giving you a frown or a gathered look around your lips? Makeup will not cover these no matter how much you apply! Shake it off, shift your thinking and choose positive thoughts and a smile! Let the smile come through your eyes, as well as, the curve of your lips.

Some free gifts for you

Thank you very much for reading my book! I hope you have discovered some ageless skin secrets and have found some valuable advice to follow. I'd like to send you some more tips and tricks, along with some samples of new amazing products as I uncover them. The science of skincare is always evolving!

Visit AgelessSkinSecrets.com to receive your free tips and samples.

Did You Enjoy This Book?

Please leave an online review – it's really important for authors like me!

Other books from Iron Ring Publishing

Visit IronRingPublishing.com for the current catalog.

Lose a pants size in two weeks!

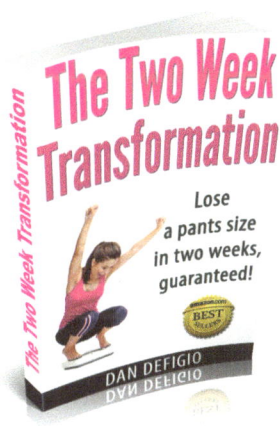

The Two Week Transformation is a simple, straightforward system that will start to change your body in just two weeks.

It's a simple guide that tells you exactly what to do for the next two weeks – what you should (and shouldn't) eat, recommended supplements, exercise tips, and some extra credit options too, if you want to really get serious.

If you follow this two-week plan exactly, you're guaranteed to lose at least one pants size, and you will feel fantastic!

Here's why you'll love The Two Week Transformation:

- It's an easy detox plan that DOESN'T involve complicated phases, measuring portions, or starving yourself

- You'll get proven nutrition secrets for maximum fat loss

- You'll be energized and feel great!

- You'll learn how to stop sabotaging yourself and finally find a way to lose weight quickly and easily

Get the kickstart you've been waiting for, and start your Two Week Transformation right now at TwoWeekTransformation.com.

Also available in Spanish!

Keeping Romance Alive

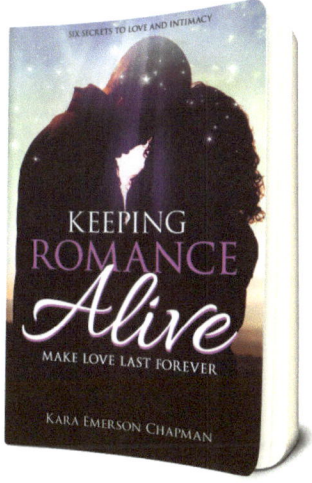

Keeping Romance Alive delivers the secrets to lasting love and intimacy in a committed relationship.

In this book, you'll find:

- Warning Signs That Your Relationship Is In Trouble
- Keeping Your Love Tank Full
- What Drives Men – What Men Seek In a Relationship
- What Drives Women – What Women Seek In a Relationship
- Being Vulnerable vs Being Needy
- Avoiding Jealousy and Resentment
- What Drives Couples Apart
- 6 Ways To Keep Love Alive

- Effective Communication

** Also included is a handy list of **101 simple romantic idea**s you can start using right now!

Get your copy at IronRingPublishing.com.

About the Author

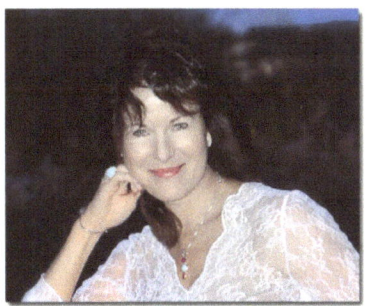

Paula Hawley is a holistic wellness consultant and an avid information-gatherer who is committed to guiding clients towards high-quality foods, safe and effective supplements, healthy lifestyles, and helping people achieve ageless and radiant skin. Paula is a veteran massage therapist specializing in healing bodywork and homeopathy. She also makes some great music:

Great Skin: Aginginreverse.nerium.com
Great Hair: Aginginreverse.mymonat.com
Music: PaulaHawley.com

www.ingramcontent.com/pod-product-compliance
Lightning Source LLC
Chambersburg PA
CBHW050818290526
45792CB00001B/164